T0126430

the little book of
NUTRIENTS

Published by OH!
20 Mortimer Street
London W1T 3JW

Disclaimer:
The information contained herein is for general information and
entertainment use only. The contents are not claimed to be exhaustive,
and the book is sold on the understanding that neither the publishers
nor the author are thereby engaged in rendering any kind of professional
services. Nothing contained in this book should be construed as or
intended to be used for medical diagnosis or treatment, or any other
purpose whatsoever. Readers are encouraged to confirm the information
contained herein with other sources and review it carefully with their
appropriate, qualified medical or other appropriate service providers.
Neither the publishers nor the author shall have any responsibility to
any person or entity regarding any loss or damage whatsoever, direct
or indirect, consequential, special or exemplary, caused or alleged to be
caused by the use or misuse of information contained in this book.

ISBN 978-1-91161-093-9

Editorial consultant: Sasha Fenton
Editorial: Victoria Godden
Project manager: Russell Porter
Design: Ben Ruocco
Production: Freencky Portas

A CIP catalogue record for this book is available from the British Library

Printed in China

10 9 8 7 6 5 4 3 2 1

the little book of
NUTRIENTS

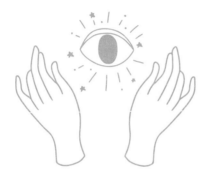

marlene houghton, PhD

CONTENTS

Nutrients are necessary for growth, for the normal functioning of the body and the preservation of life. The primary nutrients known to be essential for humans are amino acids, carbohydrates, essential fatty acids (fats), vitamins, minerals and trace minerals. We need every one of these nutrients daily to stay well. Nutrition is the process of taking in all these nutrients, assimilating and using them.

Nutrients help to build strong bones, protect us from environmental pollution and keep the skin healthy, to name just a few of their functions. They are found in everyday foods, such as vegetables, fruits, grains, legumes, meat, fish and dairy, so by following a well-balanced diet, we can provide the body with all it needs for good health. There are also some nutrient-rich, specialist sea and earth foods, but these are not in the everyday foods category, so they supplement an already healthy and varied diet. They are usually bought by health enthusiasts who want to add different and unusual foods to their diet. Often sold as supplements, they are a powerful source of added vitamins, minerals and amino acids.

"Let food be your medicine and medicine your food."

HIPPOCRATES – "THE FATHER OF MEDICINE"

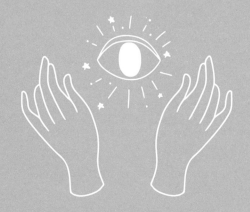

CHAPTER

1

KNOW your
NUTRIENTS

Many of us do not ingest the required amount of nutrients needed for good health due to eating unhealthy diets. Even though we in the Western world have more than enough to eat, there are still borderline nutritional deficiencies in many people. We must take every opportunity to eat foods in their unrefined state to get the most benefits from the vitamins, minerals and other food complexes they contain.

The main factors that influence nutritional status are the quality of the food, the nutrients it contains, the quantity of food we eat, the efficiency of absorption by the digestive process, and how the body utilizes the food we take in.

We should try to obtain all the nutrients we need from a variety of natural sources and make the most of nutrient power. In this way, we can be sure that we are consuming nutrient-rich wholesome food that will build good health and vitality.

Nutrients are nature's answer to radiant health. They work at a slow pace and are not like drugs that work straight away. A poorly nourished individual's health improves slowly, with the person steadily progressing towards normality. Nutrients are part of the body, so side effects are minimal.

Vitamins, minerals, amino acids and trace minerals have existed for thousands of years. Still, they were not discovered until the twentieth century, and it was only in 1911 that the first of the vitamins were identified.

Since few of these vitamins can be manufactured by the body, it is essential to our health that they are obtained from food sources.

These foods are used by whatever part of the body needs them, so if we want to stay healthy, it is up to us to provide the body with all the nutrients it needs to carry out its vital work of keeping us well.

Helpful tip

A Chinese sage once said:
"Death enters through the mouth",
and with the improvement in
nutritional science over the years,
along with the fact that nutritional
medicine is now accepted as
a valid way to avoid disease,
we see just how right this
ancient sage was!

We all know that a proper diet is essential if we want to stay fit and healthy, but many people do not know which nutrients are required daily, and in which food sources they can be found. What exactly is healthy eating?

It is actively choosing nutrient-rich foods. If we do not adhere to a healthy diet, we actually encourage health problems.

Helpful tip

The better the diet, and the richer in the nutrients, the healthier a person will be. We have all heard the mantra "you are what you eat", but you are also what you absorb. For this to happen, the diet must contain the correct nutrients for the utilization of food, and it needs the appropriate co-factors to enhance absorption.

This advice is based on that given by the *British Society of Nutritional Medicine*.

I have listed the essential vitamins, minerals, trace minerals and other food sources where these vital nutrients can be found. We can contribute to our own good health by choosing the right foods to eat in a balanced diet that contains all these nourishing and beneficial elements. If our bodies are to maximize the benefits of proteins, fats and carbohydrates, a wide range of vitamins, minerals and other factors are needed. Often these are only required in tiny amounts, but, without them, an imbalance can result.

Nutritionists believe that a diet that includes a wide variety of healthy food can provide all these essential nutrients. They also say that eating well will prevent many of the modern degenerative diseases that now afflict thousands of people.

Healthy foods that supply all the nutrients must not be underestimated.

It is sensible to increase our intake of fresh fruits and vegetables and to cut down on unhealthy fats and processed foods. When we make these changes, we notice improved health, fewer colds and more energy.

In time, it will become easier to eat healthy foods, and we won't be tempted to go back to unhealthy, devitalized foods.

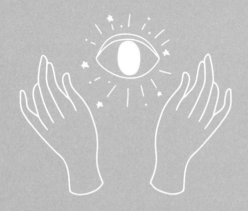

CHAPTER
2

VITAMINS and
MINERALS

Vitamins and minerals are substances that help keep our bodies in a balanced equilibrium. If this equilibrium is upset, symptoms of minor ailments can appear. Without a sufficient intake of these valuable nutrients, severe deficiency diseases can occur. A well-balanced diet will provide all the necessary nutrients that we need for health and wellness. However, finding foods that contain all the right nutrients is not as easy as people think.

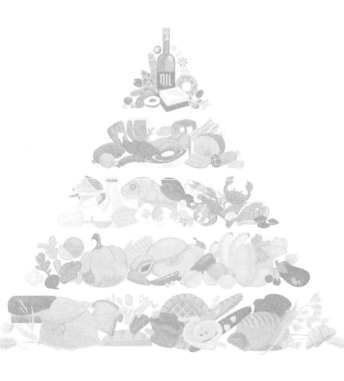

SOIL DEFICIENCY

Many foods are grown on nutrient-deficient soils, or they are imported from countries that are thousands of miles away. Often chemical fertilizers and pesticides are used to improve growth. If the earth has been overworked, chemicals are likely to have been poured into the soil by the time the foods appear on the supermarket shelves. In this way, many of the nutritious qualities that should have been in the foods are lost. Plants are only as edible as the soil they have been grown in.

Organic foods are grown without pesticides, herbicides and insecticides, and are allowed to ripen naturally. If it is not always possible to obtain naturally grown organic foods, you may need to take a decent-quality supplement. As well as eating a varied diet, this will ensure that you are obtaining all the nutrients required for good health.

VITAMINS

Vitamins are organic compounds that are essential for human growth, function and nutrition. You can only get vitamins through your diet, as the body itself can't synthesize them naturally.

The following list gives you an understanding of the particular benefits of the different types of vitamins and the various natural sources.

VITAMIN E

This vitamin occurs in two forms: retinol and the precursor to vitamin A that is called beta-carotene. The fat-soluble form, retinol, is animal-derived, and it is stored in the liver. Vitamin E supports eye health, improves immune and respiratory function and encourages cell division for normal growth.

Best sources: cod liver oil, eggs, liver, milk and butter.

BETA-CAROTENE

This pigment is found in brightly coloured fruits and vegetables. It is not technically a vitamin, but it converts into vitamin A when the body needs it. Grandmother was right when she said, "Put colour on your plate!" Vegetarians can be assured that if their diet is rich in fresh fruits and various coloured vegetables, they will not go short of this valuable nutrient.

Best sources: red, green and orange fruits, such as mangoes, apricots, blood-red oranges, tangerines, cantaloupe melon and tomatoes. Also, vegetables such as broccoli, spinach, curly kale, carrots and red peppers.

VITAMIN B COMPLEX

This is a water-soluble group of vitamins, so a constant supply is needed every day. The B complex family is made up of several nutrients. They work together in what we call synergy, but all have distinct functions.

Best sources: these valuable nutrients are found in wholegrain bread, milk, eggs, wheatgerm, brown rice and green leafy vegetables. They are also found in cheese, meat and fish.

VITAMIN B1

Ensures the proper function of the nervous system and aids the release of energy from food.

Best sources: unprocessed wholegrain cereals, wheatgerm, brown rice, beans, liver and pork.

VITAMIN B2

Strengthens hair and nails and promotes healthy skin. It also reduces stress.

Best sources: milk, eggs, liver, lean meat, green leafy vegetables and brewer's yeast.

VITAMIN B3

Promotes healthy skin, aids digestion and supports a healthy nervous system.

Best sources: lean meat, poultry, fish, legumes, wholewheat products, cheese and avocados.

VITAMIN B5

Strengthens the immune system and aids the production of energy and hormones.

Best sources: brewer's yeast, eggs, peanuts, chicken, molasses and wholegrain cereals.

VITAMIN B6

Maintains healthy skin, supports the nervous system and balances hormones.

Best sources: bananas, wholegrain cereals and wheatgerm.

VITAMIN B9

Also known as folic acid, vitamin B9 is essential for growth, reproduction and the development of a healthy baby in the womb.

Best sources: green leafy vegetables, nuts, eggs, lentils, oranges and bananas.

VITAMIN B12

Regulates healthy blood cells and the immune system.

Best sources: liver, eggs, milk, blue cheese, beef and fish.

BIOTIN

Not an actual vitamin, but plays a role in the metabolism of amino acids.

Best sources: dried beans, peanuts, egg yolks, mushrooms, cauliflowers, bananas and grapefruits.

CHOLINE

Not a real vitamin, but a key factor that complements the B complex family.

Best sources: egg yolk, lecithin, wheatgerm, brewer's yeast, nuts, pulses and oranges.

VITAMIN C

Famous for its wound-healing properties, this is also a natural antihistamine. It helps maintain healthy gums, teeth and vision and boosts the immune system.

Best sources: citrus fruits, strawberries, blackcurrants, broccoli, cabbage and potatoes.

VITAMIN D

Aids the absorption of calcium and builds strong bones and teeth. It also helps the absorption of vitamin A.

Best sources: salmon, sardines, tuna, mackerel, cod liver oil, egg yolks, milk and butter.

VITAMIN E

Strengthens blood vessels and heals scar tissue. It supports healthy skin and helps the circulation.

Best sources: unrefined vegetable oils, avocados, asparagus, almonds, green and leafy vegetables.

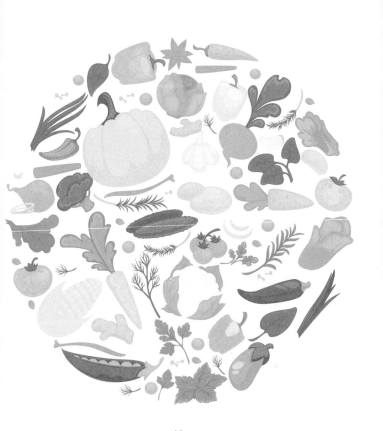

MINERALS

Minerals are inorganic substances that are major essential nutrients needed for the healthy functioning of the body. They are single chemical elements that engage in many different processes.

This following list gives you an understanding of the particular benefits of the different types of minerals and the various natural sources.

BORON

A bone-strengthening mineral that is claimed to prevent osteoporosis.

Best sources: nuts, dried fruits and root vegetables (if propagated in boron-rich soil).

CALCIUM

Builds strong bones and teeth and helps muscles to contract and blood to clot.

Best sources: dairy products, yoghurt, eggs, fish, sunflower seeds and seaweeds.

MAGNESIUM

An anti-stress mineral that reduces muscle spasms and eases pre-menstrual syndrome.

Best sources: nuts, figs, soybeans, wholegrain cereals, meat, fish and seafood.

PHOSPHORUS

Converts food into energy and combines with calcium in the bones and teeth.

Best sources: wholegrain cereals, eggs, meat, dairy products, fish, nuts and seeds.

POTASSIUM

Supports the normal heart rhythm, regulates water balance and conducts nerve impulses.

Best sources: green leafy vegetables, bananas, oranges, beans, sunflower seeds, lean meat and coconut milk.

Helpful tip

To get all your essential vitamins
and minerals, eat a varied diet with
foods from all different colour
groups to ensure you get a little
bit of everything. Vegetarians
and vegans can make up for any
elements they lack by eating a
wide cross-section of plants,
pulses and grains.

TRACE
MINERALS

We only need tiny amounts of
trace minerals to stay well, but
these micro-nutrients are as
vital to us as the major vitamins
and minerals.

The following list gives you an understanding of the particular benefits of the different types of trace minerals and their various natural sources.

CHROMIUM

Stabilizes blood sugar, improves insulin functioning and boosts immune function.

Best sources: brewer's yeast, broccoli, wholegrains, mushrooms, liver and shrimps.

COPPER

Aids iron absorption and takes part in forming red blood cells.

Best sources: wholewheat, prunes, dried beans, peas, olives, shrimps and most seafood.

IODINE

Regulates the thyroid gland and controls the body's metabolic rate.

Best sources: kelp, fish, seaweed, onions and vegetables grown in iodine-rich soils.

IRON

Important for keeping the blood healthy, as it carries oxygen around the body.

Best sources: red meat, beans, dried fruit, nuts and green leafy vegetables.

MANGANESE

Helps energy metabolism, blood sugar control and thyroid function.

Best sources: avocados, pulses, oats, almonds, hazelnuts, wheatgerm, pineapples and plums.

MOLYBDENUM

Encourages normal cell function and growth, and it also metabolizes iron.

Best sources: bread, buckwheat, wheatgerm, pulses, wholewheat pasta and legumes.

SELENIUM

Improves general immune function and is needed for the manufacture of the body's protein.

Best sources: Brazil nuts, brewer's yeast, garlic, tuna, brown rice, wheatgerm and broccoli.

SILICON

Aids the use of calcium within the bones, and strengthens the skin.

Best sources: root vegetables, brown rice, fruits and vegetables grown in nutrient-rich soil.

SULPHUR

Promotes healthy skin and helps maintain oxygen balance for proper brain function.

Best sources: lean beef, dried beans, chicken, pork, eggs, cabbage, kale, peas and garlic.

VANADIUM

Helps nutrient transport into cells, boosts energy and inhibits cholesterol formation.

Best sources: black pepper, dill seeds, parsley, spinach, mushrooms and shellfish.

ZINC

Aids tissue repair and is vital for a healthy immune system and skin.

Best sources: meat, oysters, brewer's yeast, wheatgerm, pumpkin seeds, mushrooms and eggs.

Helpful tip

Be mindful to include these trace minerals in your diet, but as humans need only small amounts of them every day, avoid taking a greater quantity than you need. High doses can result in illnesses such as gastric upset, nausea, vomiting or even more serious toxicity effects.

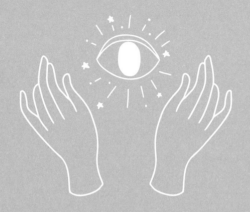

CHAPTER
3

A to Z

of AMINO ACIDS

Amino acids are chemicals from which proteins are built. They are produced in the body and found in foods.

They may play a role in strengthening the immune system and in other health-promoting activities. Nutritionists believed that a protein should be "complete", meaning that it contains all the essential amino acids in adequate quantities. Further research in nutritional science has discovered that these potent amino acids have their own individual therapeutic effect on the body's metabolism.

Amino acids are the building blocks of life. Nothing exists in nature without them, as they are the constituents of protein as well as the molecule of life, DNA.

Around twenty-two amino acids have been identified. Of these, nine cannot be made by the body, and so must be supplied by the food that we eat. The following amino acids are therefore considered essential, and each one plays a significant role in maintaining health. They are found in protein foods, including meat (chicken, game, pork) wheatgerm, oats, eggs and dairy products, especially ricotta and cottage cheese.

CYSTEINE

Needed to absorb the mineral selenium, and to protect the body from pollution and free radicals. Contains sulphur, required to create collagen and control blood sugar levels.

Best sources: turkey, chicken, yoghurt, eggs, cheese, legumes and sunflower seeds.

ISOLEUCINE

Aids skin growth, the rebuilding of muscle and healthy haemoglobin production.

Best sources: eggs, turkey, chicken, lamb, cheese, soy protein, fish and lentils.

LEUCINE

Lowers blood sugar levels and promotes rapid bone and skin healing.

Best sources: eggs, dairy products, soybeans, chicken, fish, legumes and nuts.

LYSINE

Needed for the growth and repair of tissues, and has been shown to help control coldsore viruses.

Best sources: eggs, cheese, fish, lima beans, meat, soy products, milk, yeast, nuts and seeds.

METHIONINE

Helps protect against toxic substances and destructive free radicals.

Best sources: soybeans, garlic, fish, eggs, meat, onions, seeds and yoghurt.

PHENYLALANINE

Helps control the skin's natural colour and regulates the thyroid gland.

Best sources: almonds, cottage cheese, lima beans, pumpkin and sesame seeds.

THREONINE

Regulates neurotransmitters in the brain, and may fight depression.

Best sources: poultry, lean beef, pork, soybeans, lentils, nuts and seeds.

TRYPTOPHAN

Helps induce natural sleep and reduces pain sensitivity and tension.

Best sources: bananas, dried dates, meat, whole peanuts or peanut butter.

VALINE

Regulates the metabolism and helps prevent neurological disorders.

Best sources: soybeans, cheese, mushrooms, wholegrains, meat, fish and poultry.

Helpful tip

Hot lemon and honey drinks are helpful for colds, while ginger and peppermint can ease nausea. Barley sugar or glacé mints can remedy travel sickness, and a little sugar can help ease a bad headache. Bananas help nervous exhaustion and upsetting events, while chocolate cheers you up and tea is comforting.

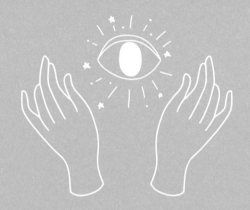

CHAPTER

4

ANTI-
OXIDANTS

Among the most powerful antioxidants are an elite group of vitamins called the ACE vitamins. They are a group of super-nutrients that are a particularly valuable addition to the diet, as they protect the body from the harmful effects of highly reactive and unstable molecules called free radicals, or oxidants.

Busy modern lifestyles, poor eating habits, smoking, stress, too much alcohol and environmental factors all increase free radicals, causing damage to the body's cells, and this may lead to a deficiency of these vital antioxidant nutrients.

This "ACE team" fights against the process of oxidation that occurs within the body.

This oxidation can be seen in everyday life. A sliced-up apple quickly oxidizes, turning brown, because it is reacting with the oxygen in the air.

The same happens in the human body; it becomes rusty, just like a car left outside and exposed to the oxygen in the atmosphere.

This is not a pretty situation when it happens in the human body, and if you want to help slow down this process, you need the ACE team.

The three key antioxidants that neutralize free radicals are vitamin A (beta-carotene, the vitamin found in plants), vitamin C, and vitamin E.

The ACE team contains vital nutrients that help slow the ageing process rather than allow it to accelerate, as so often happens when people don't have a healthy, varied diet that supplies all these cell-protectors. However, this is not all that they do.

Antioxidants protect all tissues against the damaging effects of these highly reactive and unstable molecules that can lead to many degenerative diseases and contribute to the ageing process.

These antioxidant nutrients protect the surrounding cells from damage. When the body has an adequate supply of these, they can inhibit free radical formation.

When the diet supplies ample antioxidants, the damaging effects of excess free radicals can be limited, or even prevented. These antioxidants can be obtained from natural sources such as wholesome plant foods.

The ACE nutrients are the primary antioxidants, and they can all be found in a healthy diet that includes plenty of nutrient-rich fresh fruits, vegetables and cold-pressed virgin oils like olive oil. Olive oil is high in polyphenols, which are beneficial plant compounds.

BEST NATURAL SOURCES

- Spinach is a source of vitamin A (beta-carotene) and vitamin E.

- Cabbage is a reliable source of vitamin E.

- Oranges contain carotenoids and flavonoids and are one of the best sources of vitamin C.

- Apples are also a useful source of vitamins A and C.

- Carrots, red peppers, mangoes and cantaloupe melons, as well as green leafy vegetables such as kale and spinach, are all rich in beta-carotene.

TOP 8 ANTI-OXIDANT FOODS

Scientists measure antioxidants in foods according to FRAP analysis (ferric-reducing ability of plasma). Here are the highest-rated antioxidant-rich foods:

- Dark chocolate
- Pecans
- Blueberries
- Strawberries
- Artichokes
- Goji berries
- Raspberries
- Kale

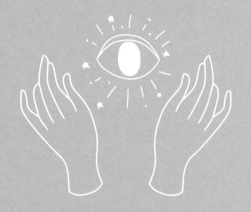

CHAPTER
5

ESSENTIAL
FATTY
ACIDS

Not all fats are bad. Essential fatty acids (EFAs) are necessary for cellular health. Those we need most are the omega-3 and omega-6 acids (named after their chemical structure).

The sea-based nutrients, the omega-3s, are mainly found in fish, fish liver oils and shellfish. This group contains EPA and DHA, the two crucial components of these beneficial oils.

There is also ALA omega-3, found in plant foods, and your body can convert ALA into EPA or DHA. Vegetarians can get some of these essential fats from plants, but they will not supply as much of these valuable oils as a fish source does. The omega-6 essential fatty acids, also considered nutritionally beneficial, are found in nuts, seeds and grains as well as some vegetable oils.

Omega-3 fatty acids play a vital role in a range of fundamental bodily processes. They cannot be made by the body and need to be supplied through the diet.

They are an essential source of energy, and they make up the protective membrane that surrounds each cell, strengthening the cell structure.

These fats produce prostaglandins, which are biological messengers that regulate a variety of body functions. They help to reduce the stickiness of the blood, making it less liable to form clots that can cause thrombosis.

Essential fatty acids have many essential functions, and the body must obtain these fatty acids through the diet or supplements. They are vital nutrients that cannot be manufactured by the body. Research has shown that they help maintain many important body functions, and if deficient in the diet, various health problems may arise.

An omega-3 deficiency can be caused by a diet too rich in red meats or poultry, or a lack of fats. It can cause skin and allergy problems, fatigue, lack of concentration, joint pain and a reduction in heart health.

In the Western diet, the omega-6 nutrients are usually over-supplied and the omega-3 under-supplied.

The omega-6 fatty acids are land-based nutrients found in vegetable oils, pulses and vegetables. We need to eat more of the omega-3 oils, as these are less present in everyday foods.

It is essential to get the right balance as too much omega-6 oil can reduce the benefits of the omega-3 oils. To get the right balance, eat more foods rich in omega-3 and reduce refined foods containing omega-6, such as polyunsaturated fats and spreads made from corn or safflower oils. Try a spread made from olive oil instead.

These vital omega-3 oils are also found in krill, which are tiny crustaceans found in the unspoiled waters of the Antarctic. These tiny creatures are an abundant source of marine nutrients, rich in EPA and DHA, and are found in superior-quality supplements.

Only a few foods are naturally high in omega-3 fatty acids. To obtain our daily requirement of these valuable oils from food, we need to eat oily fish at least twice a week. If this is not always possible, then providing the body with these fatty acids can be done by taking a decent-quality fish or krill supplement.

OMEGA-3 FATTY ACID FOODS

- Fish oil – the dark-coloured, oily fish contain the most abundant source of these essential nutrients. Herrings, mullet and rainbow trout, along with coldwater fish such as salmon, tuna, sardines and mackerel, have the highest levels of omega-3.

- Krill oil – the oil from these tiny crustaceans is easy to absorb and digest. Krill contains EPA and DHA, the essential fatty acids found in oily fish.

- Vegetarian options include linseeds, walnuts, hemp seeds, pumpkin seeds and green leafy vegetables. Non-fish sources are not as rich in EPA or DHA, but the body can convert these, although the percentage obtained may be of a low level.

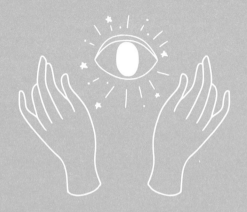

CHAPTER

6

PROTECTIVE FOOD NUTRIENTS

Nature provides us with many nutrients for extra health support. These valuable complexes are found in a wide variety of foods and are useful for specific areas of the body and various health concerns. Called "smart nutrients", they can safeguard our health in several ways. Adding these foods will introduce an extra dimension to an otherwise healthy diet, by enriching the daily intake of our usual foods with the valuable nutrients that these foods contain.

PHYTONUTRIENT FOOD GROUPS

Phytonutrients are the bio-active complexes in plants ("phyto" means plant). They are found in plants with a multi-coloured array of colours from green, orange/yellow, red, blue/purple and white. Phytonutrients support health in a variety of ways and there are substantial amounts in fruits, vegetables and grains.

Phytonutrients have not yet been proven essential but are known to offer many health benefits when included in a balanced diet.

The importance of "whole food" is well understood, as is the fact that many of the nutrients in our food work together to promote health.

That is why the daily diet should consist of a wide variety of the following nutrient-rich foods:

- **Anthocyanosides** – a flavonoid that fights free radicals and is found in red and purple fruits

- **Carotenoids** – found in fruits and vegetables with a red, yellow or orange colour

- **Flavonoids** – a large group of phytochemicals found in colourful plants

- **Phytochemicals** – substances in fruits, vegetables, grains, herbs and other plants

- **Polyphenols** – beneficial plant compounds with antioxidant properties

BILBERRY

Bilberry is highly nutritious, and it is packed with certain powerful flavonoids, which are the pigments that give bilberries their rich purple colour. These substances are believed to have a role to play in the maintenance of capillary strength. Many healthful qualities of this fruit derive from the anthocyanoside contents, which are the plant's main constituents. These protective food nutrients and health-promoting attributes are believed to help maintain eye health by supporting the circulation around the eyes.

TOMATOES

Tomatoes contain a compound called lycopene, a phytonutrient and a carotenoid that gives tomatoes and certain other fruits their red colour.

This nutrient is a significant source of the carotenoids, and it is also found in red fruits, such as watermelon, red grapefruit, guava, and tomatoes that have been cooked. Cooking helps release the valuable lycopene nutrient, which means that canned tomatoes are even better for us than fresh tomatoes.

PUMPKIN and RED PEPPERS

Pumpkin and red peppers contain the carotenoid called lutein that is necessary for healthy eyes, and lutein is known to help eye health by promoting clear vision. It does this by absorbing the sun's harmful rays and neutralizing free radicals. Lutein is also found in plentiful amounts in green vegetables.

POMEGRANATE

Pomegranate's deep red colouring comes from its flavonoid and polyphenol content. It is loaded with beneficial nutrients, it protects against free radicals, and it is rich in antioxidants. The juice of the pomegranate may support blood pressure and boost immunity.

RESVERATOL

Resveratrol is a beneficial nutrient found in red grapes and red wine. This is a rich source of polyphenols, and it is packed with antioxidants that help protect against the oxidative damage caused by free radicals. It is believed to help support healthy heart function.

TIP

Many phytonutrients have antioxidant properties that help prevent damage to cells throughout the body and are thought to reduce the risk of cancer, heart disease, stroke and even Alzheimer's. To get these, make sure you "eat a rainbow" by choosing especially dark and brightly coloured vegetables and fruits in your diet.

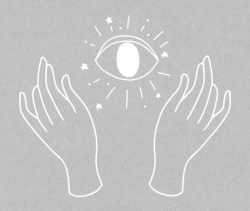

CHAPTER

7

IMMUNE-BOOSTING FOOD NUTRIENTS

A healthy immune system is critically important to help us withstand the many viruses and bacteria that surround us, and science has found that a healthy, varied diet and lifestyle is a powerful defence against germs. If we supply the immune system with the nutrients it needs to carry out essential functions, this internal army will serve us well. This immune system is a team player, and each part has its own specific task. Ideally, this marvellous defence system should be smooth-running.

Still, due to stress, illness, poor nutrition and unhealthy lifestyles, our immune system can weaken, and then our health begins to suffer. We must eat food rich in nutrients so that they can continue to protect us. Natural, organic wholesome food will provide the immune system with the nutrients it needs to function healthily and to keep it strong. The basic principle of healthy nutrition is that all nutrients work together in synergy. The interaction between nutrients forms the basis of good health.

Although many nutrients are supportive of a healthy immune system, some have a starring role in rebuilding and strengthening the immune system.

NUTRIENTS
that boost the
IMMUNE
SYSTEM

VITAMIN A

This vitamin helps to maintain strong cell walls. When we have an infection, this vitamin becomes depleted, which is when secondary infections can take hold.

If there is insufficient vitamin A, there will be fewer lymphocytes in the body, and as these form part of the immune army, those that remain will be weak and unable to fight off the infection. This vitamin is needed to help the immune system do its job of keeping the body's defences secure.

VITAMIN C

This vitamin stimulates the T and B cells, which are the part of the immune system that improves the mobility of the white blood cells (the soldiers of our immune system), which are the protectors against foreign substances.

This well-researched vitamin boosts the bacteria- and virus-killing ability of some immune cells. When bugs manage to penetrate the body, specific chemicals are activated. This can only take place successfully if there is enough vitamin C present. If the cells do not have sufficient vitamin C, they cannot digest the invading foe.

Working in tandem with this vitamin is a group of phytonutrients called bioflavonoids, which is also known as vitamin P.

BIOFLAVONOIDS

A group of phytonutrients
also known as vitamin P,
these substances are found
in nature along with vitamin
C, supporting, enhancing and
complementing its actions.
Together they work to help
maintain the health of the
immune system.

SPECIAL GROUP
of BIOFLAVONOIDS

Hesperidin, rutin, quercetin, citrin, flavones and flavonols are the best known bioflavonoids. They have been found to have specialized and added benefits in their own right.

Plants appear to increase the concentration of these nutrients in response to adverse conditions, possibly due to their antioxidant qualities. Vitamin C is more effectively absorbed when combined with bioflavonoids.

Natural sources of

VITAMIN C

and

BIOFLAVONOIDS

These are found in the pulp and rind of citrus fruits, vegetables, grapes, blackcurrants and rosehips.

VITAMIN E

This scavenger of free radicals interacts with vitamins A, C, and the trace mineral, selenium. Vitamin E is an integral part of the body's defence system.

Best sources: cold-pressed vegetable oils, especially virgin olive oil.

CAROTENOIDS

These compounds work with vitamin A and are a group of related nutrients. They are found in the most colourful plants in nature. Chlorophyll hides the carotenes that exist in dark green leafy vegetables. The deeper the green, the more carotene is present.

Best sources: green, red and yellow fruits, and green leafy vegetables.

MANGANESE

This trace mineral is vital to the body's antioxidant defence system. It helps the body use vitamins B and C. The body needs manganese to make interferon, a natural antiviral agent. Interferons are a group of proteins present in the blood all the time. When an infection penetrates the body's exterior, these antiviral interferons are activated, but only if there is enough vitamin C and manganese present.

Best sources: almonds, wheatgerm, oats, organic oatcakes, wholegrain cereals, beans, beetroot, plums and pineapples.

SELENIUM

This trace mineral is important for cognitive function and immunity, and it works in conjunction with vitamin E.

Best sources: onions and animal products.

ZINC

This trace mineral is another immune-enhancing nutrient. It is essential to over 80 body processes and helps support a well-functioning immune system.

Best sources: pecan nuts, all seeds and soy lecithin.

The vitamins and trace minerals featured in the previous pages are all found in easily accessible foods. The addition of these foods in the daily diet will help support your body's defence system, enabling it to function in tip-top condition.

All fresh fruits and berries are beneficial for the immune system, especially apricots, kiwis, avocados, blackberries and strawberries.

The best vegetables to fortify the immune system are Brussels sprouts, broccoli, kale, spinach, watercress, carrots, sweet red and orange peppers, onions and garlic.

If you can eat at least half of your fruits and green leafy vegetables raw, you will be adding a colourful array of green and rainbow power to your daily diet.

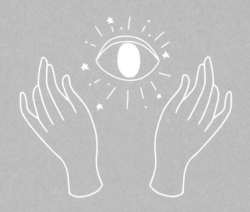

CHAPTER

8

SEA and
EARTH
FOODS

Several earth foods and kinds
of seafood may not be easily
found in supermarkets, although
you may find them in gourmet
shops or good health stores.
They are rich in nutrients,
and many people eat them to
add an extra boost to their
dietary regime.

The sea foods group consists of types of green-blue algae and the earth foods are a group of Chinese mushrooms that have been used by Eastern cultures as medicine for centuries.

Many scientific studies now support traditional health claims about the benefits of these interesting and unusual mushrooms.

ALGAE

There may be more than 25,000 species of algae in the world. Most of these algae live off sunlight or organic matter like bacteria. Seaweeds are larger micro-algae, and some are used for food.

This micro-algae, which is called phytoplankton, support all higher life in the oceans.

Blue-green algae were known to cave-dwellers and provided them with an essential source of nutrition. The ancient Egyptians consumed algae and Oriental herbalists used algae to improve vitamin deficiencies in their patients. There are even records of these nutrient-rich plant foods in the Book of Exodus in the Old Testament.

There are blue-green microalgae such as spirulina, and green algae such as chlorella. These are the two most popular ones that you can find in health shops. Another well-known seafood is Klamath algae, which comes from Lake Klamath in Oregon, USA.

These nutrients may help a healthy body work more efficiently, increasing its ability to fight off infections. This is more important than ever today, with the emergence of superbugs that are resistant to many antibiotics. Algae are natural wholefoods, which are always the best source of nutrients.

CHLORELLA

Chlorella is a green algae that is a fresh-water, single-celled plant containing several nutritious and health-building nutrients. It gets its name from the high level of chlorophyll, which is the green plant pigment that it uses to make energy from sunlight.

Chlorella contains a higher level of chlorophyll than any other plant. Also, it is a reliable source of vitamins, minerals, antioxidants, omega-3 fatty acids, fibre, amino acids, and enzymes.

Full of healthful compounds, chlorella packs a nutrient punch. It has strong cell walls that must be broken down for it to be used as a health food. During the 1970s, a method was discovered that allowed chlorella to be digested more quickly, so after this, it began to be used as a health food.

The Japanese are the world's largest consumers of chlorella supplements, and they have used them since the nineteenth century. Chlorella is believed to be an immune booster and a detoxifier.

It is available as capsules, tablets and green powders.

SPIRULINA

These microscopic blue-green algae have been used as a food for centuries, and these amazing fresh-water vegetable algae can capture the sun's energy.

Spirulina is a rich source of chlorophyll, it is filled with vitamins and proteins, and it is the most abundant source of mixed carotenoids in the world.

Spirulina is much more abundant in organic iron than raw spinach and beef liver, and, being high in vitamin E, it supplies more of this valuable vitamin than wheatgerm.

It is a useful source of GLA, which is an essential fatty acid that the body converts into hormone-like compounds. Spirulina is sometimes included in macrobiotic and vegetarian diets.

The carefully controlled growing environments safeguard these products and make sure that only the highest-quality algae supplements reach the market. If you decide to take blue-green algae, ensure that you only use tested and approved products.

Available as capsules or tablets, in liquid form, as a tincture or a powder, you can mix it with fruit juice or include it in your favourite smoothie.

KLAMATH ALGAE

This is a unique strain of wild algae that grows in its own habitat – the cold, pristine, mineral-rich waters of Klamath Lake – and is not produced artificially. This blue-green algae is protected by the clean air and the high-intensity sunlight in which it grows.

It is believed that these algae have health-giving properties due to the antioxidant effects of their beta-carotene and chlorophyll content.

Klamath also helps populate the body's own supply of intestinal flora that is needed for the healthy function of the immune system and for optimal wellbeing.

Rich in natural antioxidants, carotenoids, organic minerals, trace elements, vitamins, amino acids, essential fats and enzymes, these nutrient-dense blue-green algae also contain vegetable protein and vitamin B12. They are suitable for vegetarians and vegans and are available in capsules or tablet form.

SUPER MUSHROOMS

There is an exclusive group of exotic-sounding mushrooms that differ from the ones you see in local supermarkets. Although they are less well known in Europe, they have a long history of use in Traditional Chinese Medicine and in Japanese culture, where they are used for their medicinal qualities.

Their medicinal use has been well documented by Oriental herbalists, and they have been treasured as remedies for disease for thousands of years.

Modern science has found that these mushrooms have specific beneficial qualities, which explains their long history of use by such ancient cultures.

These super fungi are growing in popularity because scientific studies revealed the health benefits of these ancient earth foods. They have been used for centuries as immune boosters, longevity tonics and as natural health supporters. They may be found in Asian supermarkets, gourmet shops and health stores.

It sounds strange, but this species of mushroom is challenged by the same viruses and bacteria that humans are, and this has enabled them to develop the same defences as the common enemies that afflict mankind.

Four of these mushrooms are particularly valuable when it comes to helping us to stay well.

CORDYCEPS

Cordyceps are known as the "longevity mushroom", as they are traditionally used in China to support wellbeing and to help the body build strength and endurance. They are also reputed to be good for the lungs.

Cordyceps are rich in manganese, zinc, selenium and potassium.

MAITAKE

Maitake is known as the "dancing mushroom". It has been used for centuries, due to its immune-enhancing effect, which is believed to be related to the mushroom's content of polysaccharides. These are sugar-like components of many cells that stimulate the immune system.

Maitake mushrooms are rich in lipids, vitamins B1, B2 and D, and eight amino acids.

SHIITAKE

Known as the "samurai mushroom", shiitake contains the phytonutrient lentinan, which has beneficial properties for the liver and supports a healthy immune system.

Shiitake mushrooms are rich in B-glucans, B vitamins, lipids, four amino acids, calcium, magnesium, manganese, iron and zinc.

REISHI

Known as the "mushroom of immortality", reishi has traditionally been used to boost *qi*, which is a vital energy force of the body. It has a high antioxidant content, so it has been used historically to support the immune system.

Reishi is rich in iron, zinc, magnesium, manganese, calcium and potassium.

These mushrooms are available as:

- Dried and fresh produce
- Capsules and tablets
- Liquids
- Powders
- Tea

The addition of any one of these algae
or super mushrooms to your daily
programme will add another group
of valuable foods that are believed
to have significant benefits for
maintaining health and fighting illness.

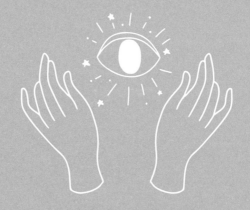

CHAPTER

9

PROBIOTICS

Probiotics are found in foods that are believed to add extra health benefits to the general standard nutrients found in everyday foods. They are called functional foods. Many long-lived societies have attributed cultured dairy drinks with gut-friendly probiotics for their long life and general good health. Probiotic means "for life", and it relates to the healthy bacteria found in the gut, which keeps us well.

In the gut, there is an entire ecosystem made up of different bacteria, yeasts and fungi, living and working harmoniously, unless the ecosystem is disturbed, and the harmful bacteria begin to proliferate. If that happens, it sends the immune system into overdrive, causing inflammation and undermining health. When we are healthy, the friendly bacteria that inhabit the gut work to keep the body in check and help to maintain our health.

However, stress, processed food, antibiotics and illness all reduce the number of beneficial bacteria in the gut. The immune system is our body's natural defence system, and it guards us against bacterial infections. Still, few people are aware that most of this happens in the gut.

Probiotics form a line of defence against toxins and the harmful types of bacteria that reduce the number of friendly bugs in the digestive tract during times of stress, infection and illness.

The friendly micro-organisms in probiotics populate the gut and help maintain a good balance of the right type of bacteria that is important for immune health. When the gut is brought back into balance, the beneficial bacteria will support the immune system in its job of protecting us.

These protective strains have several functions, including:

- Affecting the pH (acidity or alkalinity), creating an optimum ecosystem

- Preventing unhealthy bacteria and fungi from colonizing the gut

- Helping the absorption of vitamin K and several vitamin Bs

- Aiding the absorption of iron and calcium

- Inhibiting the overgrowth of harmful bacteria, fungi and viral organisms

Plain, "live" yoghurt contains friendly micro-organisms, lactobacillus acidophilus and bifidobacteria that make this a healthy addition to the diet. There are many more of these sub-strains of these micro-organisms being discovered, and each one has a different function.

The idea is that if you regularly eat probiotic foods, have dairy drinks or take supplements, you will outweigh the harmful bacteria in the gut with the good ones, keeping both the digestive system and the immune system in good health.

Prebiotics are separate from probiotics. They are indigestible plant fibres that work alongside probiotics to increase the good bowel bacteria. They also enhance the colonic environment, helping the friendly bacteria to proliferate and continue to populate the gut for a more extended period, thus improving intestinal health.

Prebiotics are the type of fibre that occurs in fruits and vegetables. They are found naturally in foods such as leeks, onions, asparagus, chicory (salad leaf), Jerusalem artichokes, garlic and bananas. You can boost the number of beneficial bacteria in the gut naturally by eating a diet rich in these healthy foods.

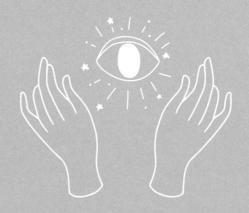

CHAPTER
10

SUPER-GRAINS and SEEDS

Grains or cereals are possibly the most important staple food of all, and they have been the main foods of many cultures for thousands of years. In very ancient times, cereal grains gradually became more critical than meats that were hunted, fish that were caught or fruits and nuts that were picked. Wheat was baked into bread, and this was called the "staff of life".

The staple grain varied according to the location. In the West, wheat and rye were most valued, followed by oats, barley and millet. Rice and millet were the staples of the East.

Today these divisions no longer exist, and grains are the primary source of energy for many people throughout the world.

GRAINS

Grains are loaded with protein, fibre, vitamins and minerals. Grains should be whole, and flours should be made from the whole grain.

Grains provide two types of fibre: soluble and insoluble. Insoluble fibre is concentrated in the bran, and soluble fibre can aid weight loss, partly because it helps rid the body of toxic waste.

Soluble fibre is soft and gluey, and it absorbs water. Insoluble fibre does not absorb water. Both types of fibre are essential in the diet. Research links fibre with the prevention of life-threatening diseases. The American Dietetic Association suggests that high-fibre foods can reduce the risk of chronic diseases.

Grains are an excellent source of complex carbohydrates, which fuel the body's energy needs and provide this energy in a time-released way. These valuable grains also contain essential vitamins, minerals and phytochemicals, so they offer an assortment of weapons that help the body fight diseases.

Whole grains are full of goodness and should be included in the daily diet, replacing the refined grains that are found in many products.

Many grains that are eaten in other cultures were pretty much unknown in the Western world, but this is changing, and several types can now be found in supermarkets.

AMARANTH

Amaranth is a staple of the ancient Aztec culture, but it isn't technically a grain. Flour made from amaranth can be used for making crackers, cookies and flatbreads.

Key nutrients: protein, calcium, fibre, B vitamins, magnesium, zinc and iron.

Phytochemicals: phenolic compounds function as antioxidants to protect cells.

BARLEY

This was the most important grain of the ancient Greeks, Romans and Hebrews. Today it is used in bread, vegetable soups, such as Scotch broth, and stews. Whole hulled barley is the most nutritious.

Key nutrients: fibre, magnesium, manganese, vitamin E, B-complex vitamins, zinc, iron and calcium.

Phytochemicals: tocotrienols function as antioxidants and beta-glucans are powerful immune enhancers.

BUCKWHEAT

This grain is sometimes called "Saracen's corn", as it was brought to Europe from Asia by the Crusaders. It is not a grain in the botanical sense, because it is related to sorrel and rhubarb. Its value lies in its rutic acid content, which is a complex plant substance.

Key nutrients: iron, almost all the B-complex vitamins, vitamin E, fibre and calcium.

Phytochemicals: rutin has a beneficial effect on the circulation.

BULGUR WHEAT

This ancient wheat product has continued to exist in Eastern Europe. It is made from wheat that has been parboiled, then dried, and then the whole wheat kernels are cracked. It is a rich source of antioxidants and fibre. Bulgur wheat can be used in soups, salads, stews, casseroles and pilafs.

Key nutrients: protein, fibre, potassium, choline, B vitamins, iron and calcium.

Phytochemicals: phenolic compounds and anti-inflammatory properties.

MILLET

This was possibly the first cereal grain to be used, and it became a staple food in China even before rice was introduced.

It is still an important staple in many parts of the world and, except for quinoa and amaranth, millet is the most complete protein of any grain. The whole grain can be added to homemade granola and bread.

The Hunza, a remarkable people who are known for their longevity, eat as part of their diet chapatti bread made from wheat-millet, buckwheat or barley flour. The flour is whole and not refined, nor does it have the germ removed. The germ has astonishing nutritive powers, which must contribute to the Hunza's good health.

Key nutrients: protein, fibre, iron, calcium, magnesium, B vitamins and manganese.

Phytochemicals: includes lignin, a protector against disease, and phenolic compounds.

OATS

Oats have been used since the time of the Roman Empire. They are a reliable source of complex carbohydrates and are also high in protein. Oats are the best grain-source of calcium and many other minerals. All types of oats are useful as a breakfast cereal or in muesli and granola.

Key nutrients: manganese, phosphorous, copper, vitamin B, selenium, magnesium and zinc.

Phytochemicals: tocopherols and tocotrienols function as antioxidants and beta-glucans.

QUINOA

Quinoa was called the "gold of the Incas", and it has been eaten in South America for thousands of years. This fashionable grain has gained popularity because of its high nutritional value. Known as a super-grain, it provides all the amino acids and is gluten-free.

Key nutrients: fibre, magnesium, vitamin B, iron, potash, calcium, phosphorous and vitamin E.

Phytochemicals: phenolic compounds, antioxidant and anti-inflammatory.

RICE

Nearly half the people in the world eat rice as their staple. Wholegrain rice is rich in complex carbohydrates, and it is low in fat and calories. There are many types of healthy, speciality rice in health food and gourmet shops, and these can be used to prepare ethnic dishes.

Key nutrients: protein, fibre, calcium, magnesium, iron, B vitamins and manganese.

Phytochemicals: lignin.

RYE

Rye has been cultivated for nearly 2,000 years, and by the Middle Ages, rye had become the staple grain throughout Europe. Dark rye bread with its distinctive flavour is eaten in Germany, Russia and Scandinavia. It is dense and filling, and it is used in bread and crackers. Whole rye can be cooked as a cereal.

Key nutrients: protein, fibre, B vitamins, calcium, magnesium, manganese and zinc.

Phytochemicals: phenolic compounds and lignans.

SPELT

This ancient grain is more than 5,000 years old, but it is enjoying a revival. It has a sweet, nutty taste, and is rich in all the essential amino acids. Spelt contains many nutrients that have a stimulating effect on the immune system.

Key nutrients: protein, fibre, B vitamins, iron, manganese, vitamin A, calcium and potassium.

Phytochemicals: lignin.

WHEAT

Wheat is one of the world's most important cereal crops, and it is one of the oldest grains. Whole wheat, where the bran and germ are intact, is nutritionally superior to wheat that has had the bran and germ removed. Whole wheat is high in insoluble fibre, which is a protector against intestinal problems.

Key nutrients: protein, fibre, iron, B vitamins, vitamin E, magnesium and manganese.

Phytochemicals: tocotrienols, beta-glucans and lignin.

SEEDS

There are several useful kinds of seeds, some of which can be nibbled as a snack, and others that are included in food products.

FLAXSEED

This was prized by the ancient Egyptians, who used flaxseeds for food. These nutty-flavoured seeds can be added to bread, muffins and other baked goods. High in omega-3 fats, fibre and high-quality protein, they supply a wealth of health benefits.

Key nutrients: protein, fibre, calcium, iron, vitamin C, B vitamins, vitamin E and selenium.

Phytochemicals: lignans function as antioxidants.

PUMPKIN SEEDS

In China, the pumpkin is called the "emperor of the garden". The seeds are an excellent source of essential fatty acids and are richer in iron than any other seed.

Key nutrients: protein, fibre, magnesium, manganese, zinc, selenium, vitamin A, vitamin C and vitamin E.

Phytochemicals: phytosterols, immune enhancers and protectors against disease.

SESAME SEEDS

In Hindu mythology, the God Yama blessed the sesame seed. These seeds are packed with vitamins and minerals, and high in iron. They are used in African, Chinese, Indian and Turkish cuisines.

Key nutrients: vitamin A, B vitamins, vitamins C and E, manganese, magnesium and selenium. They also contain lecithin, inositol and choline.

Phytochemicals: phytosterols enhance immunity and protect against many diseases.

SUNFLOWER SEEDS

These were first found in the Western plains of North America, and they are a member of the daisy family. Crisp, crunchy sunflower seeds are a nutritious addition to breakfast cereals, baked goods and salads.

Key nutrients: these are rich in B-complex vitamins, magnesium, selenium, iron, calcium, vitamin C and vitamin E.

Phytochemicals: tocopherols and lignans function as antioxidants.

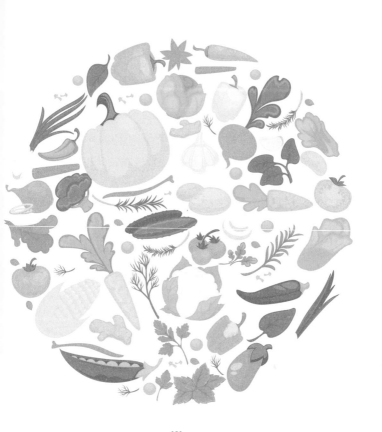

CONCLUSION

Your diet is a powerful tool to the maintenance of your health and the prevention of disease. Throughout the book you will have discovered the nutrients that are the most important to include in your daily diet, the food sources they are found in and how they can help you and your family.

Good luck with your cooking and eating, and with the pleasure you will get from trying a wide variety of nutrient-rich foods.